THE PROSTATE CANCER ESSENTIALS FOR SURVIVAL SERIES

DOSIMETRY AND RADIOTHERAPY FOR PROSTATE CANCER

MICHAEL J. DATTOLI, MD

WITH SPECIAL CONTRIBUTIONS BY JONE FAY, RT, CMD

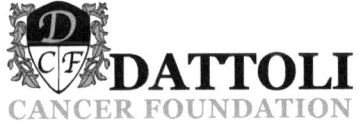

SARASOTA, FLORIDA

Dosimetry and Radiotherapy for Prostate Cancer: Precision Treatment Design for DART, IMRT, and Brachytherapy

Copyright © 2018 by Michael J. Dattoli, M.D.

All rights reserved. No part of this work may be reproduced or transmitted in any form or by any means, electronic or mechanical, including photocopying or recording, or by any information storage or retrieval system, except as may be expressly permitted by the 1976 Copyright Act or in writing by the publisher.

ISBN-10: 1-983597-27-9
ISBN-13: 978-1-9835-9727-5

Published by the Dattoli Cancer Foundation, Sarasota, FL
Imprint of record: CreateSpace, Charleston, SC
Book design and composition by Dan van Loon, Batavia, IL

MEDICAL DISCLAIMER

This booklet is intended as a supplement but not as a substitute for the medical advice of a physician. It is imperative that you consult a qualified healthcare professional with regard to all matters relating to your health and particular situation. Neither the publisher nor the authors bear responsibility for any consequences due to the reader's decision to use any particular treatment, medication, dietary supplement or other healthcare practices discussed in this book.

DEDICATION

This booklet is dedicated to all those whose lives have been touched by prostate cancer, and to the patients and their families whom we are privileged to serve and educate as cancer care providers.

ACKNOWLEDGMENTS

We are deeply grateful to a number of people who have contributed to this booklet in a number of ways. Our thanks to Greg Lawrence, for his editorial efforts and to Ginya Carnahan, Chris Wells, Jennifer Undella, MLT, ASCP, and Chris Keeler for their ongoing assistance. For her special contribution to this booklet, we are also indebted to Jone Fay, RT, CMD, a board certified medical dosimetrist at the Dattoli Cancer Center & Brachytherapy Research Institute.

We appreciate all of those wonderful patients and family members who have contacted the Dattoli Cancer Foundation for counseling and guidance and in turn have given us their support and encouragement. It is your spirit and commitment in confronting this disease that inspires us all.

CONTENTS

INTRODUCTION
Precision Radiation Therapy and Prosatate Cancer 7

OVERVIEW—IMAGING, PLANNING, AND HISTORICAL PERSPECTIVE
Diagnostic Imaging Techniques and DART–4D IG-IMRT Treatment Planning 11
Brachytherapy Treatment Planning 13
Historical and Practical Perspectives: Dosimetry and Treatment Planning 14

APPENDICES
A: Deciding What is Best for You 27
B: Glossary of Medical Terms 29
C: The Warning Signs of Prostate Cancer 43

About the Authors 44
The Dattoli Cancer Foundation Mission 45
Order More Booklets in the Series 46

INTRODUCTION

PRECISION RADIATION THERAPY AND PROSTATE CANCER

From our earliest studies of the family of diseases we call cancer and the discovery of radium just over 100 years ago, researchers have been challenged to harness and accurately focus the dual cure-or-kill power of radiation. In the century since Marie and Pierre Curie first described the radioactive properties of pitchblende, much has been learned and a great deal of medical progress has been made. In the most recent decade, the escalation of knowledge about prostate cancer has been extraordinary, and our ability to safely treat prostate cancer patients with radiation has made it the treatment of choice in a variety forms for a majority of patients.

For the treatment of prostate cancer patients, many years were required to design techniques for accurately delivering a radiation dose deep into the abdomen without damaging the important structures surrounding the prostate gland, such as the bladder and rectum. The strategy with radiation therapy over the years has been to deliver higher and higher doses more and more accurately to destroy the targeted cancer, while sparing healthy adjacent tissue in order to avoid rectal and urinary complications. Today our ability to identify minute areas of tumor within the prostate where cells are just beginning to mutate into cancer, and our skill in taming and aiming radiation has turned this therapy into an effective, reliable tool in the fight against this potential killer. It has been a welcome and timely evolution. No longer do men have to risk surgical mutilation and side effects in hopes of a possible cure.

Advancing knowledge and perfecting non-surgical treatment for prostate cancer is what the Dattoli Cancer Center & Brachytherapy Research Institute is all about. Dedicated to the treatment of prostate cancer as our only focus, we are not content to merely cruise along in the mainstream of the field. Our pioneering physicians are committed to exploring new horizons, to asking tough questions and challenging the "old school" practitioners who believed that radical surgery was the "gold standard" for treating prostate cancer. In the process we are saving more men's lives than ever before, and equally important, we are safeguarding their quality of life after treatment. Our commitment to providing only leading edge, state-of-the-art radiation therapy is deeply rooted in who we are—and why our Center has earned the reputation it enjoys.

The purpose of this booklet is to help you understand how treatment planning and dosimetry calculations are carried out with advanced radiation therapies such as brachytherapy (seed implantation) and Dynamic Adaptive Radiotherapy (DART) utilizing all of the modalities associated with 4-Dimensional Image-Guided Intensity Modulated Radiation Therapy (4D IG-IMRT). Preparation for radiation therapy is a rigorously complex process that involves exact determination of the region to receive treatment and the appropriate dose of radiation. For patients and their loved ones, knowing what to expect during the treatment process is one of the keys to fighting this disease.

As members of the Dattoli Cancer Team, our shared goal with this booklet is to help you make *informed decisions* as you consult with your doctor. We strongly advise you not to delegate your decisions to someone else. After all, it's your body and your health that are at stake. As you gather information, always consider the source and use your own judgment about your personal needs. *You will know best what is right for you.* Don't be afraid to voice your concerns to your doctor and don't hesitate to ask questions—you have every right to know the answers and to expect a standard of care with which you are entirely satisfied.

—*Michael J. Dattoli, M.D.*

OVERVIEW

IMAGING, PLANNING AND HISTORICAL PERSPECTIVE

Diagnostic Imaging Techniques, DART and 4D IG- IMRT Treatment Planning

By the time we meet most of our patients, they have already had an initial diagnosis, so the process begins with additional laboratory work and more definitive diagnostic exams. Day One with Team Dattoli begins with our advanced 3-D color-flow Doppler ultrasound. During the diagnostic process, we use this imaging technique to pinpoint the location of suspicious tissue within the prostate gland. Dual monitors allow our patients to see exactly what the doctor is seeing. The color-flow Doppler ultrasound allows us to discern areas of abnormal blood flow (vascularity) that are indicative of a tumor site.

A one-of-a-kind computer program then allows us to view the Doppler images in 4 dimensions (the fourth is motion), rotating the image 360 degrees to reveal the most complete picture of the gland possible. Knowing the location and extent of tumor in the gland is the first critical piece of knowledge necessary to perform an accurate biopsy and to build an effective treatment plan.

Another major diagnostic tool is the helical CT scan. This modality gives us three dimensional views of soft tissue. The CT scan helps us to precisely locate the prostate and surrounding structures. This tool enables us to create a computerized simulation of the patient's gland and its intimately located structures, including the bladder, rectum, seminal vesicles, nerve bundles and lymph nodes. These are all considered when designing a treatment plan for the patient. This CT scanner is also outfitted with a QCT program that performs a bone density exam of the patient. It is important to learn the status of the patient's bone integrity before any treatment begins. QCT scans are repeated following treatment to determine if any bone degradation has occurred.

The initial CT scans will be reviewed by a physician and a treatment strategy will be mapped out. Once the diagnostic procedures are complete, we turn to the Dosimetry Suite, where a detailed treatment plan will be developed, tailored to the unique individual needs of each patient. This is accomplished through what we call an *inverse planning* process, utilizing the information that was taken during each patient's initial scan. The doctor draws on the structures on the CT scan that will be critical during planning. All of that information is entered into computers in the Dosimetry Suite in order to facilitate the planning process.

Today the CT scan is often combined or fused with other sophisticated imaging and diagnostic modalities, such as multiparametric MRI and Dynamic Contrast Enhanced MRI (DCE-MRI). These fused imaging modalities represent the state of the art in imaging and have greatly enhanced our ability to diagnose and treat the disease.

Our dosimetrists are able to see critical structures in a three-dimensional image of the patient's body, first rendered from the CT scan. Those structures include the prostate gland, the bladder, the rectum, the seminal vesicles, and the lymph nodes. All of these structures are important in the treatment planning process, as some organs such as the bladder and rectum will receive only a limited dose of radiation, while other structures such as the prostate, seminal vesicles and nodes will receive a higher dose in order to effectively eradicate the cancerous tissue. Dattoli Cancer Center certified medical dosimetrist Jone Fay will further explain and illustrate this process later in this booklet.

Once the dosimetrists have identified the structures in the three dimensional view, they are able to place the radiation beams on the CT scan, so that they can see the exact position of the linear accelerator and path of each beam that will deliver the radiation, how the machine will deliver the dose, and what the dose looks like in the patient's body. For a particular treatment, they typically place on seven fields of radiation. They start with a field from the top, another field from the right side, and others from the right back side, from the left side, back and front. Once the beams are placed, the computer will do a complex calculation process that will produce what are called isodose lines. These lines show exactly what the dose will look like as it goes through the patient's body. Any spots that are hot or cold are identified, and the treatment is customized to each patient.

Once the plan has been completed in the treatment planning computer, the parameters of the treatment can be checked before it goes to the treatment machine. One of the parameters is the multileaf collimator that actually shapes the radiation beam during each treatment. The movement of the leaves can be viewed exactly as they would perform on the machine during treatment.

Once the treatment is completed on the planning computer, the plan will then be validated by the on-staff physicist, using a separate computer software program that is able to analyze the treatment to be sure that everything is correct. At that point, the plan is sent over to the treatment unit and the patient is ready to begin radiation therapy.

DART and 4D IG-IMRT treatments using this uniquely formulated plan will usually begin within three or four days after the initial diagnostic exams. The standard protocol at our institution calls for 4 to 4 ½ weeks of daily radiation treatments. Each plan is actually developed as four cycles. The second and third cycles are more focused to deliver the radiation beamlets more tightly on the prescribed area.

Brachytherapy Treatment Planning

If a patient's treatment calls for brachytherapy, our team of medical dosimetrists and physicists will create a three-dimensional map for the placement of the radioactive seeds. Using color-flow Doppler ultrasound images, the doctor will designate the areas that he wants treated, including the prostate gland and usually a margin of tissue around the gland. At that point, the ultrasound images are entered into the computer system. The prostate can be viewed in slice by slice cross-sections through the gland, adding the radioactive materials (seeds) along the way. Analyzing the patient in this fashion with ultrasound, CT scans, MRI images, and so forth, and with the knowledge of exactly where the cancer is, focus can be placed on putting the radioactive materials into that tissue. This is how we arrive at the optimal plan to treat each patients individually.

Once this phase is completed, the plan is reviewed in two dimensions, moving through the gland from the anterior to the posterior, looking at all the areas, making sure there are no hot spots. Then the plan is evaluated in three dimensions, noting that the seeds are specifically loaded in a peripheral pattern, with seeds placed in extracapsular locations as needed, to minimize the dose to the urethra and penile bulb while maximizing tumor doses. The plan is reviewed by the doctor, and at that point, the seeds are ordered from Theragenics Corporation in Buford, Georgia. The seeds are shipped overnight to Sarasota Memorial Hospital. Once they arrive, a dosimetrist calibrates them, and then takes them to the operating room, where they are sterilized and ready for implantation the following day.

The day after seed implantation, the patient will return to the Dattoli Cancer Center for another helical CT scan to confirm the count and placement of the seeds and to calculate the dosimetric dispersion of the Palladium-103 isotope over a three month period. At this point, it is determined through physics calculations if the patient will benefit from additional IMRT radiation treatment to the periprostatic tissue. If indicated, supplemental treatment plans for 3 to 10 additional treatments will be developed. These post-implant IMRT treatments are usually scheduled about 3 months after the seeding procedure, at the first follow-up visit.

The palladium-103 seeds that are used have a half life of only 17 days. That means their strength is diminished by half every seventeen days. The impact of the seeds begins to peak at three weeks, and usually subsides significantly by three months. The seeds eventually become inert and remain in the body. Follow up appointments are made for 3 to 6 months and 1 year to monitor progress, with PSA, color-flow Doppler ultrasound, CT scans of the pelvis and abdomen, and other laboratory tests as indicated. By the second follow up visit, the vast majority of our patients have returned to normal lives without significant side effects.

Historical and Practical Perspectives: Dosimetry and Treatment Planning

This section is based on a presentation by Ms Jone Fay, RT, CMD, who is board certified in medical dosimetry, x-ray and radiation therapy. She has been working in the radiation field for more than thirty years and at the Dattoli Cancer Center & Brachytherapy Institute for more than nine years.

I am going to discuss dosimetry and radiation treatment planning from a historical perspective in order to appreciate how this field has changed over the past couple of decades with all of the technological progress that we have seen. One of the most striking features that I want to point out is the time that is required to do treatment planning. Years ago when I first started, it would take a week or two weeks to create a complicated plan. Now, with the aid of computers and advanced technology, we can complete complicated plans in about twenty minutes.

To proceed with this discussion, I want to define some of the basic concepts in this specialized field. Dosim-

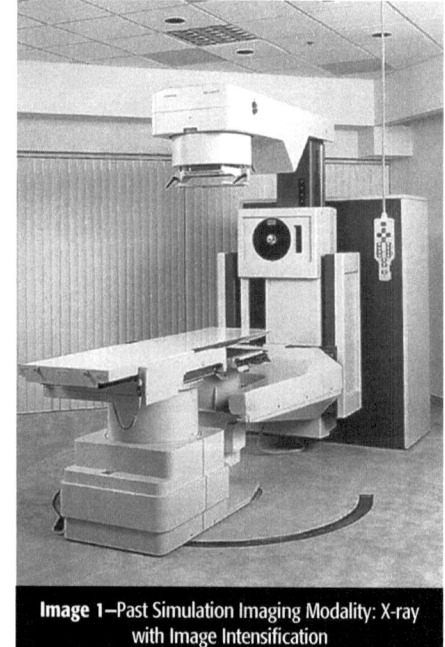

Image 1—Past Simulation Imaging Modality: X-ray with Image Intensification

etry involves the calculations, measurements and related activities required for determining the radiation dose to be delivered during treatment. These calculations are undertaken by a medical dosimetrist, who is a member of the radiation oncology team, with specialized knowledge of the treatment machines and related equipment. The dosimetrist helps implement the procedures commonly used with brachytherapy and with advanced external beam therapy such as 4D IG-IMRT. In collaboration with a medical physicist and radiation oncologist, the dosimetrist possesses the education and expertise required to generate radiation treatment plans.

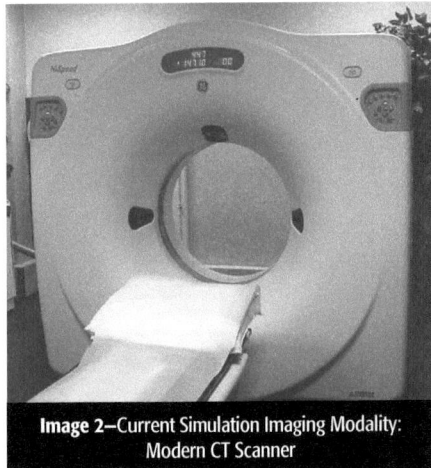

Image 2—Current Simulation Imaging Modality: Modern CT Scanner

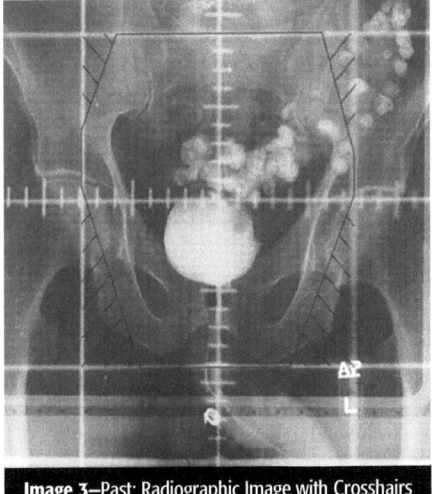

Image 3—Past: Radiographic Image with Crosshairs and Delineator Wires

Essentially, in order to come up with an individualized treatment plan, I take into account all of the information from the patient's CT scan, the doctor's initial dosimetric and target prescription, and the mechanical capabilities of the treatment machine. I sometimes describe being a dosimetrist as something akin to Frankenstein, in that like him we are made up of different parts. In fact, we play a number of roles. We are part physician, part physicist, part nurse, and part radiation therapist.

I want to illustrate how things used to be in this field and how they are now in terms of the technology and protocols that are utilized. I have to include a disclaimer here, pointing out that some of the past technology that I'm about to discuss, even though it is outmoded, is still being used by some medical centers. By contrast, at our institution we take great pride in having only state-of-the-art equipment.

Image 1 shows an x-ray table, with an x-ray tube and an image intensifier underneath. This is the kind of treatment simulation equipment that was used in the past. It was set up geometrically in the same way as the modern linear accelerator and gave

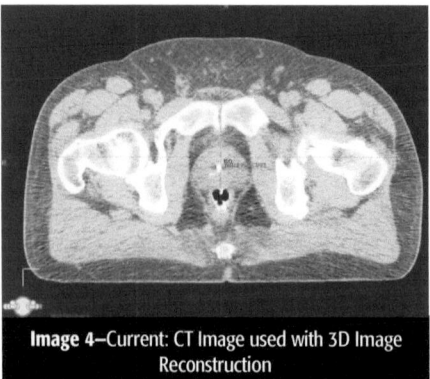

Image 4—Current: CT Image used with 3D Image Reconstruction

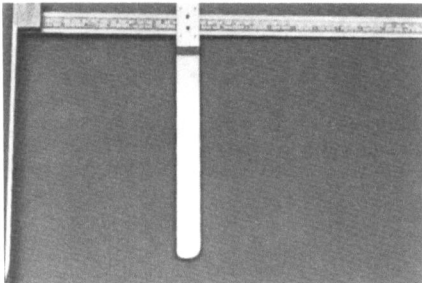

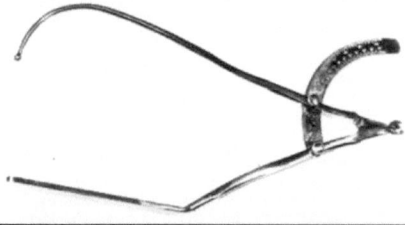

Images 5 and 6—Calipers

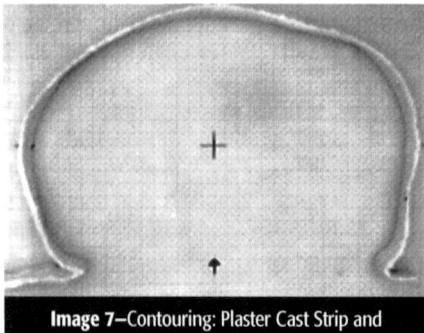

Image 7—Contouring: Plaster Cast Strip and Graph paper

plane films with a front view and a side view, or a specific angle. There was a grid pattern projected on the film that would enable us to map out a simulation field.

Image 2 shows a modern helical CT scanner. We are now able to combine CT scans with other imaging techniques such as PET (positron emission tomography) scans and MRI (magnetic resonance imaging). We use these imaging modalities in treatment planning and they enable us to better visualize the internal organs.

Image 3 shows the radiographic image of the whole pelvis, which is the way the prostate was treated years ago, when doctors could only irradiate the entire pelvic area. You can see the bladder, which has dye in it, and the colon, which also has dye in it. The simulator projected wires that delineated the area we wanted to treat. The darker hatch marks in the image are the areas the doctor wants blocked, or shielded from the radiation. It should be noted that conventional x-rays don't lend themselves to a 3-dimensional view of internal organs.

Now we have CT scans (Image 4) that enable us to discern the contour of the body in greater detail, allowing us to see how large the patient is front to back and side to side. We can also see how the prostate gland is positioned relative to the bones. The CT scan gives us more information than an x-ray, where we can only tell approximately where the prostate is. We couldn't really use the x-ray image efficiently in the computer without using other equipment, such as calipers and other contouring devices. (Images 5 and 6), Calipers are used to determine the size of various body parts. The therapist can measure width and thickness from front to back in centimeters. Calipers may look a little menacing, but they are basically just glorified rulers.

In the old days, after measuring the body parts of interest with the calipers, the dosimetrist would create a contour using graph paper and a plaster cast strip to show the outline of the body (Image 7). Prior to CT scans, the dosimetrist had to input everything by hand. The measurements were taken with calipers after the radiographic films to determine where the center of treatment would be. A plaster strip or solder wire would be placed around the patient to determine the shape of the area of interest, and then transferred to the graph paper. This process was fairly tedious and primitive, without allowing us to see the internal structures. In a sense, operating in the blind to some extent, we would transfer the shape into the computer and start the treatment planning.

Image 8 shows another contouring device called a pantograph, which is also set up to work with graph paper. A stylus would be run over the patient's body to transfer the shape onto graph paper.

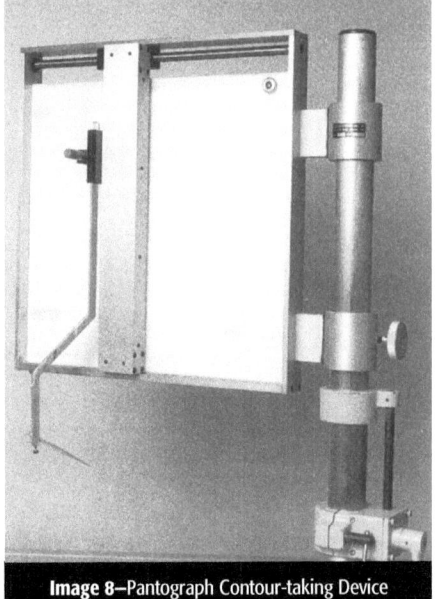
Image 8—Pantograph Contour-taking Device

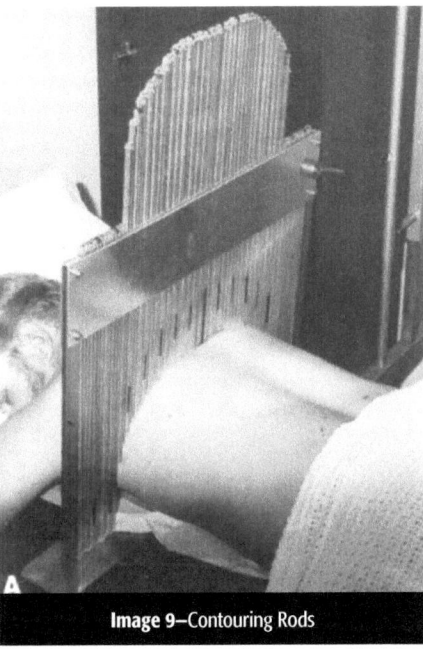
Image 9—Contouring Rods

More elaborate devices were also employed such as contouring rods (Image 9). With this technique, a bank of aluminum or steel rods would be positioned over the patient, and they would slide up and down to map the contour of the area of interest. The dosimetrist would then transfer the shape to graph paper (Image 10).

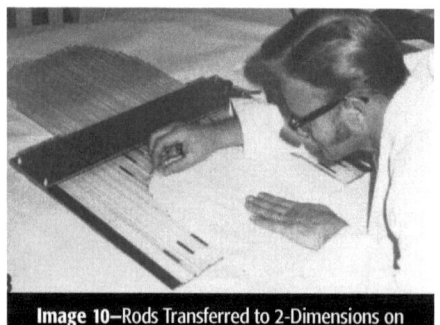

Image 10—Rods Transferred to 2-Dimensions on Graph Paper

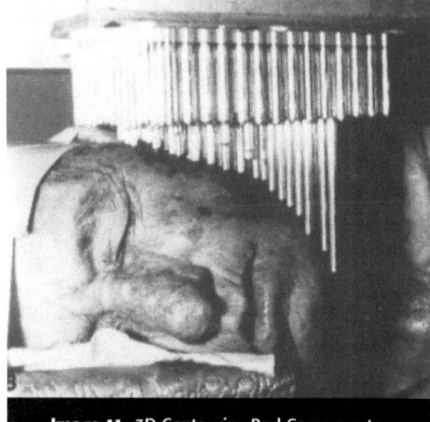

Image 11—3D Contouring Rod Compensator

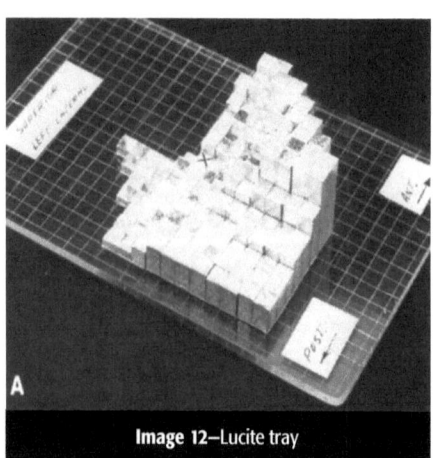

Image 12—Lucite tray

Image 11 shows a 3-dimensional rod bank device that would be used for the head and neck areas, which have a lot of contours and shape changes that need to be taken into account when directing the radiation beams. Where the chin is the thinnest, the rod is the longest. The contours could then be transferred to a Lucite tray (Image 12), where there were brass cubes that could be stacked up to reflect the shape rendered by the rods. This was actually a very crude form of what we call intensity modulation, where the radiation oncologist can adjust the intensity of the beams to fit a specific target area.

As a source of radiation, the use of Cobalt machines has become obsolete and they are no longer used in most places. A cobalt machine would utilize a radioactive cylinder of metal that was located inside the machine in a large protective housing. The Cobalt produced radiation through its decay. In the case of modern linear accelerators, we use electricity to produce photons of radiation. At the Dattoli Cancer Center, we employ the most advanced external beam technology, 4D IG-IMRT to achieve DART, which currently defines state-of-the-art in the field.

In order to treat effectively, we need to know what the radiation looks like as it goes through the body, and to accomplish that, we utilize what are called *isodose curves*. These curves allow us to measure what percentage of the dose is going to what particular depth as the radiation passes through the body. The template of these isodose curves is drawn onto the contours that were measured earlier (see

Images 13 and 14). The curves represent percentages of the original dose of radiation being delivered through the body. Wherever the isodose curves intersect, they are added together. So two 70 percent lines combined would be 140 percent. The dose is measured in centigray (cGy), what used to be called a "rad." A typical daily dose of external radiation may range from about 180 to 200 cGy.

In the past, once we had the graph paper showing the contour and we added on the templates showing the isodose radiation curves, we had a fair idea of what the radiation looked like as it went through the body, but we didn't yet know what it was doing to the target organ. After CT scans came along, we were able to more accurately visualize the structures within the body, without having to rely on graph paper and guesswork. Image 14 shows how much radiation is going to the spinal cord at the

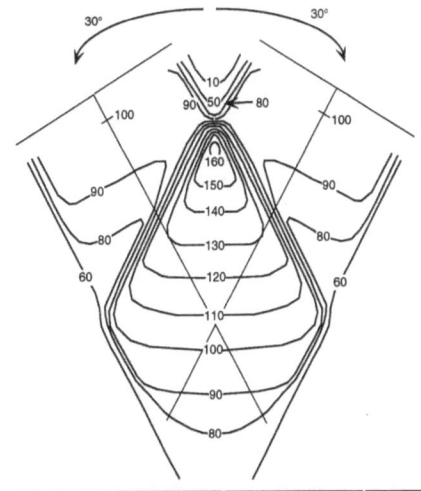
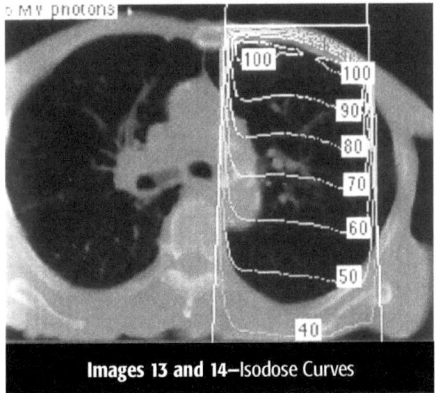
Images 13 and 14—Isodose Curves

center and to the right and left lungs. The CT scan allows us to see in 3 dimensions exactly what is happening at the tumor area and proximate tissue. The imaging is even more enhanced with PET and MRI fusion techniques.

Years ago the thinking was that the whole pelvis needed to be treated. We treated front, back, right and left sides. This was known as the 4 Field Box technique. There were a lot of side effects because the bladder and bowel were in the way and received unwanted radiation. Patients also suffered a great deal of fatigue. Of course, twenty-five years ago we didn't have more sophisticated techniques like Intensity Modulated Radiation Therapy or Conformal Radiation Therapy. Once Conformal Radiation Therapy was introduced in the 1990s, the thinking on prostate cancer changed, with the prospect of not having to treat the entire pelvis at least for a certain percentage of patients.

With Conformal Radiation Therapy, as shown in the two views of Image 15, the area of treatment is smaller. In the lateral or side view on the right, you can see

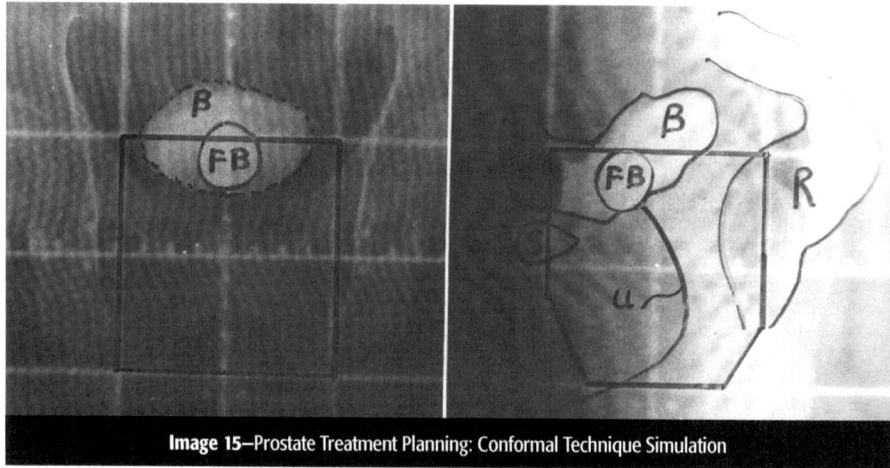

Image 15—Prostate Treatment Planning: Conformal Technique Simulation

the bladder, the rectum, and bulb of the catheter. While not visible in this image, the prostate sits right at the base of the bladder. With the Conformal approach, the entire pelvic area was no longer being treated. With a smaller area of treatment, radiation was more easily tolerated, with fewer side effects. We were able to direct the beams from multiple angles, so we were able to focus more effectively on the prostate area, while sparing areas like the bladder and rectum. This also enabled us to increase the dose to the target area, so we had greater tumor control.

In Image 16, the therapist is creating a shielding device. She has a simulation x-ray, and the physician has drawn on the image where he wants the radiation blocked out. Using Styrofoam and a hot wire, she would make a mold and pour in a molten metal alloy called Cerrobend, a mixture of lead, bismuth, tin and cadmium. The metal would cool and it would then be mounted on to a Lucite tray and put into the head of the treatment machine to focus and control the area of treatment (Image 17). Within the treatment machine there were collimators, large depleted uranium leaves that would move back and forth, right and left. This would allow the radiation therapist to design a square or rectangular field, but when you had a curved area to treat, this block design did not closely conform to the target area. Today, with IMRT, we have multi-leaf collimators that do all this for us, replacing the old fashioned shielding blocks.

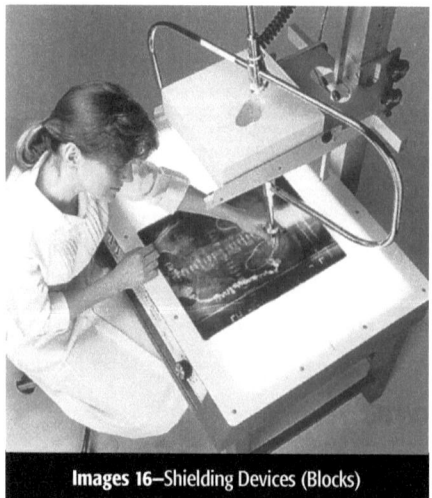

Images 16—Shielding Devices (Blocks)

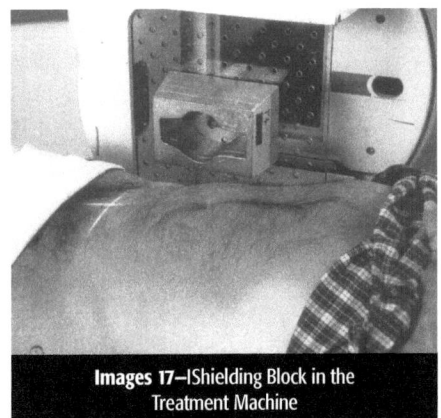

Images 17—Shielding Block in the Treatment Machine

What we do now is enter the shape into the computer, and the computer aligns the leaves of the collimator to make the beams conform to that precise shape. So our work as dosimetrists and therapists has become very refined, resulting in custom tailored plans fitted to each individual patient.

With the Conformal approach, dosimetrists would plan a 7 to 9 field approach on a treatment, and each field would have a different shielding block. The therapist would be in the room lifting these blocks up into the machine, and these blocks could weigh up to thirty pounds, taxing work for the therapists.

Image 18 compares the three techniques. The 4-field box utilizes fields from the front, back, right and left. Conformal Radiation utilizes a greater number of smaller beams. IMRT can have as many as 7 or even 8 fields, or as little as 3 fields. The fields are the angles to which the treatment machine is directing the radiation. You can see with each evolution, the target area has become more refined, while eliminating unnecessary radiation doses to the surrounding tissues.

With IMRT, we typically start with 7 fields during the first phase of therapy, which usually consists of ten treatments. In that initial phase, the treatment margin

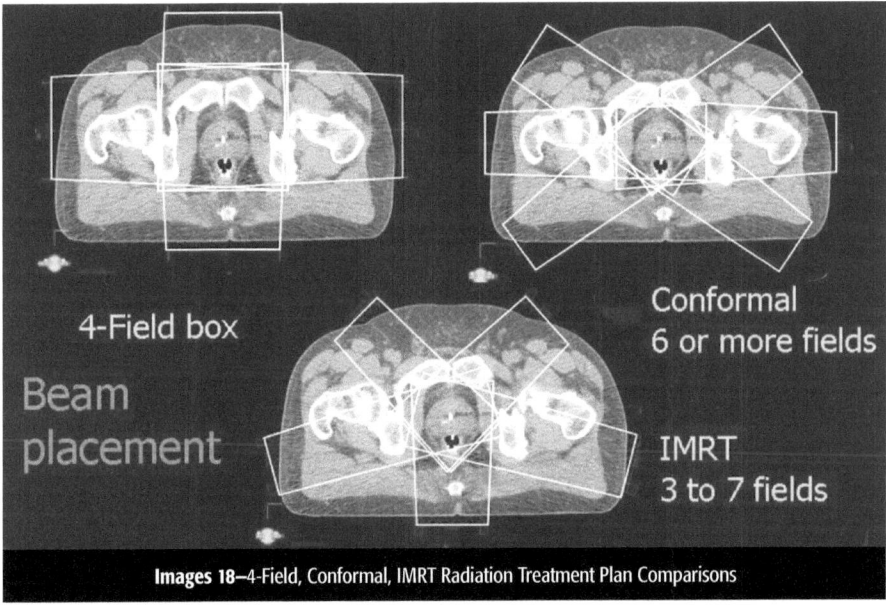

Images 18—4-Field, Conformal, IMRT Radiation Treatment Plan Comparisons

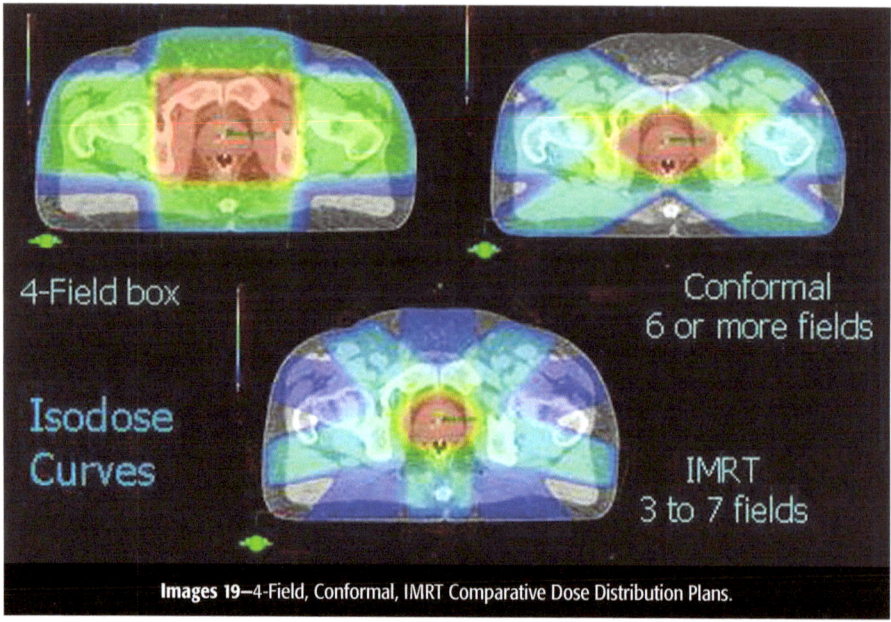

Images 19—4-Field, Conformal, IMRT Comparative Dose Distribution Plans.

is approximately 1 centimeter around the prostate target area, which includes the seminal vesicles. During the second phase of treatment (the next 10 treatments), we utilize 6 fields and a treatment margin of about ½ centimeter around those structures of interest. In the third phase, we use six fields and a margin of approximately 3 millimeters, and the fourth phase over the lymph nodes only. The prostate will be further treated by seeds, but the dose from the seeds does not reach the nodes. Therefore, the fourth phase is designed to bring up the dose level to the nodes.

Until the mid-1980's, the maximum dose that could be safely administered to the prostate was thought to be 7000 cGy. Higher doses at that time were associated with an unacceptably high risk of complications. With the improved technologies in use today, doses of greater than 8000 cGy can be safely administered and have proven more effective at killing cancer.

With the combined treatment protocol of IMRT and brachytherapy, after the patient undergoes the seed implant procedure, if indicated, he will return for a brief follow-up course of IMRT treatments that will typically utilize 4 fields.

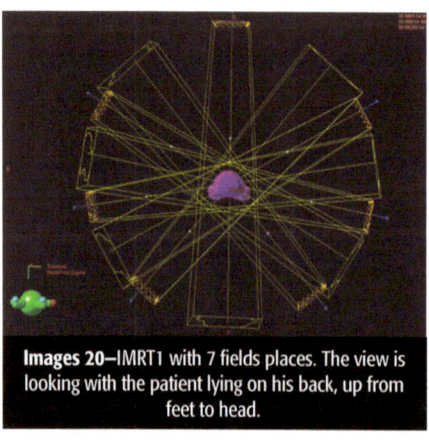

Images 20—IMRT1 with 7 fields places. The view is looking with the patient lying on his back, up from feet to head.

Image 19 shows the dose distributions, with the red area being the hotter area of radiation. The IMRT modality is able to focus and "cone" down the radiation such that it is confined to the prostate target area, thus greatly reducing side effects as compared to both the 4-Field Box and Conformal Radiation techniques.

With IMRT, we are also able to spare the urethra, concentrating the radiation in the peripheral areas where the tumors are and avoiding irritation to the urethra. The nerve bundles and penile bulb are also spared in order to preserve erectile function. Some structures in the body are more resistant to radiation than others. For example, nerves tend to be less sensitive to radiation. Normal cells and cancer cells differ in how they respond to radiation. Normal cells have a greater tolerance and ability to repair after being exposed to radiation. When the cancer cells die after treatment, they are simply eliminated from the body.

Image 20 shows the volume of interest (target) for the first phase of IMRT planning (IMRT1) with the 7 fields placed, and the target at the center of the image. We call this the "Ferris wheel."

Images 21 and 22 illustrate brachy-therapy planning. After a patient finishes the course of IMRT radiation, he will then have an ultrasound study in order to prepare for the seed implant. When planning the implant, we obtain a strip of ultrasound images, delineating the prostate, and the doctor will have drawn on the target area that he wants treated. We use a standard grid pattern template, so when we start

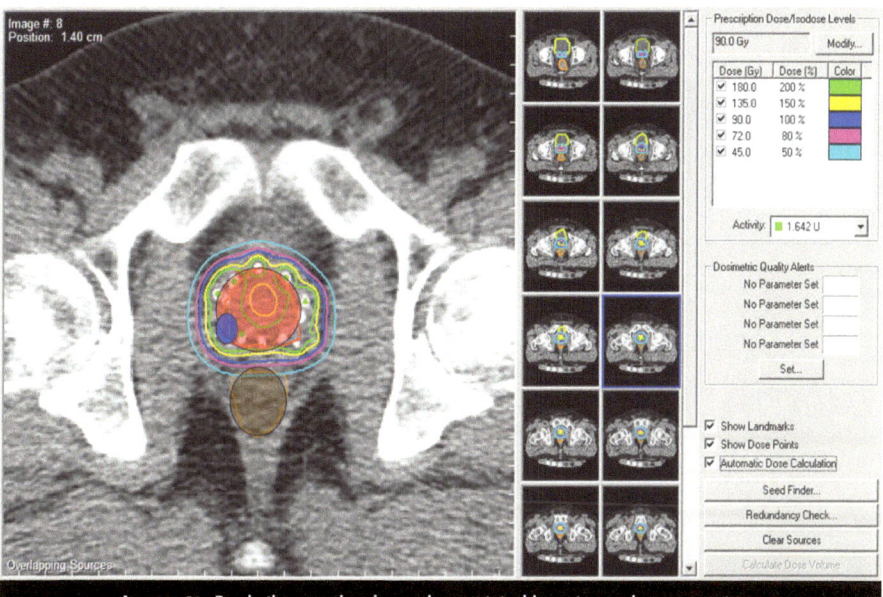

Images 21—Brachytherapy planning: red = prostate, blue = tumor, brown = rectum, white markers with green dots are the seeds.

PROSTATE CANCER ESSENTIALS FOR SURVIVAL: DOSIMETRY AND PROSTATE CANCER RADIOTHERAPY

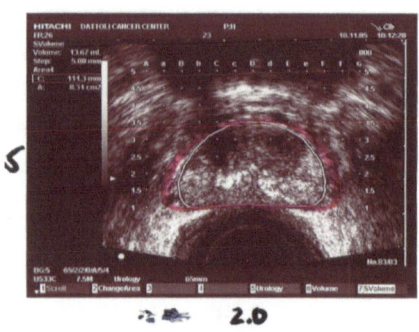

2.0
3.0

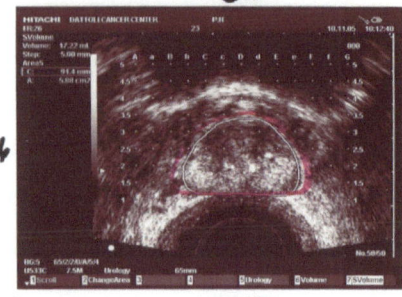

2.5

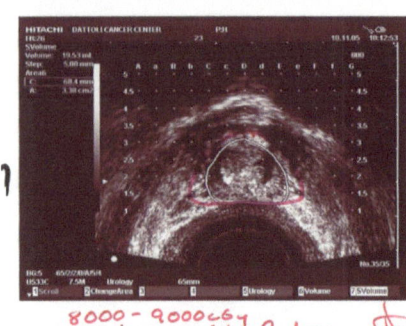

8000 - 9000 cGy
minimum peripheral dose

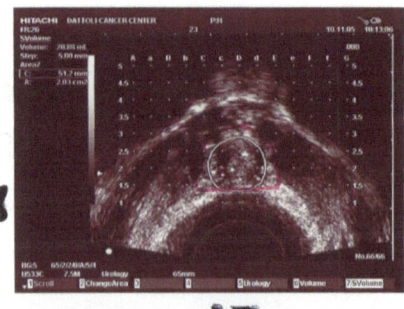

3.5

Images 22—Ultrasound strip of the prostate outlined in white with the margin drawn in that the doctor wants to implant. The grid pattern is shown.

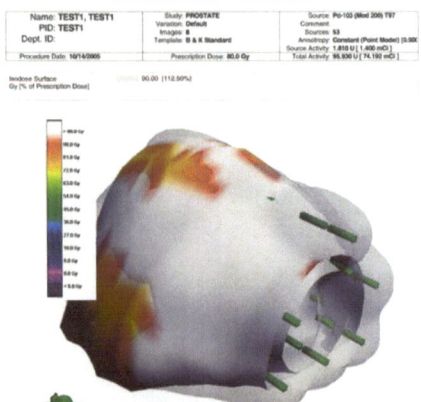

Images 23—3D view of the implant plan. The seeds are represented by green bars.

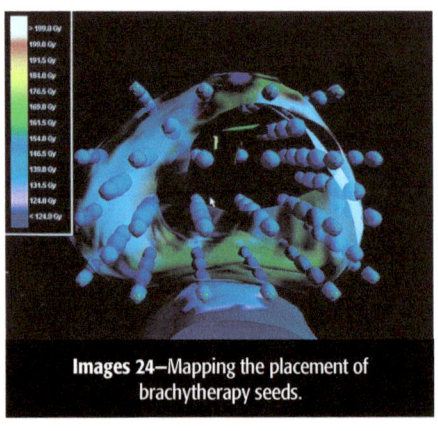

Images 24—Mapping the placement of brachytherapy seeds.

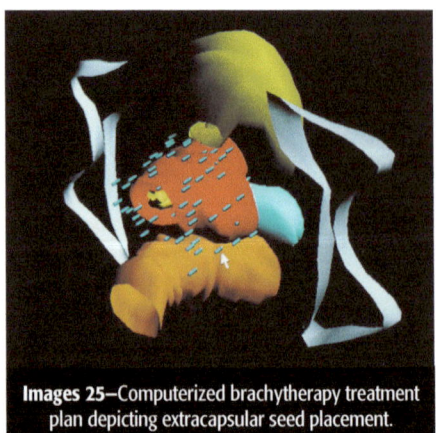

Images 25—Computerized brachytherapy treatment plan depicting extracapsular seed placement.

designing the seed placement plan, we can communicate in the operating room exactly where the seeds need to go.

This treatment plan will be translated in the Operating Room. A template will be placed over the perineum and it will have the exact same grid pattern used for designing the seed-placement plan. We also prepare a pre-plan study in order to know how many seeds we will need to order. Once in the O.R., the doctor will make the actual determination of where and how many seeds will be inserted based on the prepared placement plan, having the option of using seeds of two different strengths. He will make sure that the prostate receives a substantial dose while sparing the urethral tissue, the nerve bundles and penile bulb. We are able to accomplish that precise targeting and dose modulation because tumors in the prostate usually occur around the outer peripheral edges, which will receive a much higher dose of radiation than the interior areas and structures we want to protect. Images 23, 24 and 25 show the seed placement in 3-dimensional views of the brachytherapy plan.

The day after the implant, the patient returns to our center for a CT scan to confirm the placement of the seeds. In the body, after the seeds are implanted, they may not stay in the symmetrical pattern of the original loading plan because the body moves and the prostate will shift to some degree. We do what is called a post-plan that shows exactly how the seeds were placed and what the radiation dose distribution looks like, which will be evaluated by the doctor.

Those dosimetric calculations and the patient's disease history will be used to determine if additional IMRT treatments are indicated. If so, a supplemental treatment plan for 3 to 10 additional treatments will be generated, and the patient will return for those approximately 3 months after the seeding procedure, thus completing his therapy. Thereafter, he will be monitored, returning for a comprehensive evaluation at 3 months, six months, and then annually.

References:

Moss-Cox *Radiation Oncology* 6th Edition, Mosby 1989

Levitt, Kaplan, Potish Levitt and Tapley's *Technical Basis for Radiation Therapy: Practical Clinical Applications* 2nd Edition, Lea & Feberger 1992

Bentel: *Radiation Therapy Planning,* Second Edition, McGraw Hill 1996

APPENDIX A

DECIDING WHAT IS BEST FOR YOU

Consult with your physician, and by all means, obtain second and third opinions whenever possible, preferably from physicians with different specialties. If you have already been to a urologist, it is worthwhile to visit a radiation oncologist or medical oncologist (those with experience with hormones and chemotherapy).

Join a support group such as US TOO!, or PAACT. If you belong to any of the computer on-line services, check out the medical and health bulletin boards and mailing lists for the latest information and announcements for prostate cancer patients. Keep your personal plan of action updated.

What to Remember

- Obtain all of the advice and counsel that you can, but keep in mind that the decisions are ultimately yours to make.

- Be positive—if you have been properly staged and treated, the odds are in your favor on not having a recurrence.

- If you should have a rising PSA over time after initial treatment, don't panic. Get further tests, and if appropriate, get a biopsy, preferably guided by color flow Doppler ultrasound.

- The secret to success with prostate cancer is catching the disease early, and that is also true for recurrence.

- If testing confirms cancer, learn all you can about your options. Get second and third opinions. Become informed and empowered. Become involved with solving your problem. It's your life and body. Go for it!

- Life is full of problems and challenges. Solve this problem like any other big problem:
    1. Identify the problem.
    2. Get all the facts to confirm that you have a problem.
    3. Learn what options are available to you and weigh them carefully.
    4. Choose a qualified doctor who is experienced and with whom you are comfortable.
    5. Initiate and follow through with the solution.
- Don't be afraid to ask for help from your spouse or partner, from your family and your friends. It is more important than ever for you to turn to loved ones to get the emotional and spiritual support you need. This disease can be a difficult struggle for us, but we are not alone, and our mental attitude, prayers and our fighting spirit really can make all the difference.

To be a cancer survivor, you must first be a cancer fighter!

APPENDIX B

GLOSSARY OF MEDICAL TERMS

3D-CRT (3-Dimensional Conformal Radiation Therapy): See Conformal Radiotherapy.

5-alpha reductase (5-AR): an enzyme that converts testosterone to dihydrotestosterone (DHT).

Adenocarcinoma: A cancer originating in glandular tissue. Prostate cancer is classified as adenocarcinoma of the prostate.

Adjuvant: An additional treatment used to increase the effectiveness of the primary therapy. Radiation therapy and hormonal therapy are often used as adjuvant treatments following a radical prostatectomy. Compare Neoadjuvant.

Agonist: A chemical substance that combines with a receptor on a cell and initiates an activity or reaction. See LHRH analogs.

Algorithm: A step-by-step procedure for solving a problem or accomplishing some end, especially by a computer.

Analog: A man-made chemical compound that is structurally similar to one produced naturally by the body. See LHRH analogs.

Anastomotic stricture: narrowing, usually by scarring, of an anastomotic suture line.

Androgen: A hormone that produces male characteristics. See testosterone.

Androgen ablation therapy: A therapy designed to inhibit the body's production of testosterones.

Androgen-dependent cells: Prostate cancer cells which are nourished by male hormones and therefore are capable of being destroyed by hormone deprivation (also known as androgen-sensitive cells).

Androgen-independent cells: Prostate cancer cells which are not dependent on male hormones and therefore do not respond to hormonal therapy (also known as androgen-insensitive cells).

Anesthetic: A drug that produces general or local loss of physical sensations, particularly pain. A "spinal" is the injection of a local anesthetic into the area surrounding the spinal cord.

Aneuploid: Having an abnormal number of chromosomes, as revealed by ploidy analysis. Aneuploid prostate cancer cells tend not to respond well to androgen deprivation therapy (ADT).

Angiogenesis: The body's formation of new blood vessels. Some anti-cancer drugs work by blocking angiogenesis, thus preventing blood from reaching and nourishing a tumor.

Antagonist: A chemical substance in the body that acts to reduce the physiological activity of another chemical substance.

Anti-androgens: Drugs such as Casodex that block the activity of androgens produced by the adrenal glands at the cellular receptor sites. Androgens can block or neutralize the effects of testosterone and DHT on prostate cancer cells.

Antibody: A protein produced by the body that counteracts the toxic effects of a foreign substance, organism, or disease within the body.

Antigen: A foreign substance such as a virus or bacterium that causes an immune response or the formation of an antibody.

Antineoplastic: Inhibits growth and proliferation of cancer cells.

Antioxidants: Any substances which delay the process of oxidation in the body.

Apoptosis: The normal molecular mechanism which governs the life span of cells so that they die in a very organized way. Cancerous cells are resistant to normal apoptosis.

Benign: A non-cancerous condition. See also Benign Prostatic Hypertrophy.

Benign Prostatic Hypertrophy (BPH): Also called Benign Prostatic Hyperplasia, BPH is a non-cancerous condition of the prostate that results in a growth of tumorous tissue and increase in the size of the prostate.

Biopsy: A procedure involving the removal of tissue from the body of the patient. Removed tissue is typically examined microscopically by a pathologist in order to make a precise diagnosis of the patient's condition.

Bone scan: An imaging technique used to detect bone metastases, which appear as "hot spots" on the film. It is far more sensitive than the conventional x-ray.

BPH: See Benign Prostatic Hypertrophy.

Brachytherapy: A form of radiation therapy in which radioactive seeds are implanted into the prostate to deliver radiation directly to the tumor. Also referred to as seed implantation, or seeding.

Cancer: A cellular malignancy typically forming tumors. Unlike benign tumors, these tend to invade surrounding tissues and spread to distant sites of the body.

Carcinoma: A malignant tumor made up chiefly of epithelial cells, or those cells that form the lining of an organ or cavity. See Adenocarcinoma.

Castrate Range: The level of the body's testosterone after orchiectomy (also referred to as castration). This is the range or level, which is used by physicians as a point of comparison for those drugs, which attempt to decrease the testosterone level.

CAT Scan (or CT Scan): See Computer Tomography.

cGy: Abbreviation for centigray; a unit of radiation equivalent to the older unit called a "rad."

Chemotherapy: The treatment of cancer using chemicals that deter the growth of cancer cells.

Collimator: A device that organizes radiation such that only parallel rays or beams emanate.

Combination Hormonal Therapy (CHT): Also referred to as Combined Hormonal Blockade (CHB), or Combined Androgen Deprivation Therapy (ADT). The preferred term is ADT, often designated with a number referring to the number of agents used (i.e., monotherapy ADT, ADT2, ADT3). This combined therapy can utilize a number of mechanisms, including surgical or medical ADT, anti-androgens, 5-alpha reductase inhibitors, estrogenic compounds, agents that block adrenal androgen production, and agents that decrease the receptivity of the androgen receptor.

Combination Therapy: Refers generally to any combination of treatment modalities used to treat prostate cancer.

Computer Tomography: Computer generated cross-sectional images of a portion of the body. Also called CT or CAT scan.

Conformal Radiotherapy: A radiation treatment conforming precisely to the size and shape of the prostate, with the use of computerized planning and state-of-the-art imaging techniques. 3-Dimensional Conformal Radiation Therapy (3D-CRT) utilizes this sophisticated approach to treatment planning, as does the even more advanced Intensity Modulated Radiation Therapy (IMRT).

Cryosurgery (also referred to as Cryotherapy or Cryoablation): The freezing of tissue with the use of liquid nitrogen or Argon gas probes. When used to treat prostate cancer, the cryoprobes are guided by transrectal ultrasound.

Cytokine: Any of a class of immunoregulatory substances that are secreted by cells of the immune system.

DHT (dihydrotestosterone): The active form of the male hormone, testosterone, produced after testosterone is transformed by an enzyme known as 5-alpha reductase.

Diagnosis: Evaluation of a patient's symptoms and/or test results, with the intent of identifying and verifying the existence of any underlying disease or abnormal condition.

Digital Rectal Examination (DRE): A procedure in which the physician inserts a gloved, lubricated finger into the rectum to examine the prostate gland for signs of cancer.

DNA (Deoxyribonucleic Acid): A complex protein that is the carrier of genetic information that determines the physical development and growth of living organisms.

Doppler Ultrasound Technique: A machine that sends out ultrasonic waves that pick up the velocity of blood flow through the veins and are transmitted as sound to make an image.

Doubling Time: The time it takes for a tumor or cancerous focus to double in size.

Downsizing: The use of hormonal therapy or other forms of intervention to reduce tumor volume prior to primary, curative treatment.

Downstaging: The use of hormonal therapy or other forms of intervention to lower the clinical stage of prostate cancer prior to primary, curative treatment.

Ejaculatory Ducts: The tubular passages through which semen reaches the prostatic urethra during orgasm.

Ejaculation: The release of semen through the penis during orgasm.

Endorectal MRI: Magnetic resonance imaging of the prostate gland using a probe inserted into the rectum. Dynamic Contrast Enhanced MRI is the most effective form of magnetic resonance imaging.

Enzyme: A chemical substance produced by living cells that causes chemical reactions to take place while not being changed itself.

Erectile Dysfunction (also referred to as ED or impotence): The loss of ability to produce and/or sustain an erection sufficient for intercourse.

Estrogen: A female sex hormone that can be used as a form of therapy to inhibit the production of testosterone in patients diagnosed with prostate. cancer.

External Beam Radiation Therapy (EBRT): A form of radiation therapy that utilizes radiation delivered by an external source (machine) and directed at a target area to be radiated. In contrast to EBRT, brachytherapy utilizes radiation sources (seeds) that are internal, implanted in the target tissue. EBRT may use conventional photons, protons, neutrons or electrons.

Extracapsular Extension: Used to describe prostate cancer that has spread outside the prostate gland.

False Negative: An erroneous negative test result. For example, an imaging test that fails to show the presence of a cancer tumor later found by biopsy to be present in the patient is said to have returned a false negative result.

False Positive: A positive test result that mistakenly identifies a state or condition that does not in fact exist.

Feraheme (Ferumoxytol): A ferromagnetic nanoparticle which is taken up by normal macrophages with the lymph nodes.

Fistula: With regard to prostate cancer, an abnormal passage due to injury or disease that connects an abscess or hollow organ to the surface of the body or to another hollow organ. If there is significant damage to the rectal wall proximate to the bladder, a fistula may occur between the bladder and rectum.

Flare Reaction: A testosterone surge caused by the initial use of an LHRH analog, causing a temporary increase of tumor growth and symptoms (known as clinical flare), or an increase in PSA (biochemical flare).

Foley Catheter: A catheter inserted in the penis and threaded through the urethra to the bladder where it is held in place with a tiny, inflated balloon. It removes urine from the bladder and can be used to irrigate the urethra and prevent blood clots.

Free PSA: PSA that is unattached to any major protein in the blood. Free PSA is associated with benign prostate growth. The percentage of free PSA is derived by dividing the free-PSA level by the total-PSA x 100. Studies have show that men with free PSA % > 25% were at low risk for prostate cancer, while men with PSA % < 10% were at high risk for having prostate cancer.

Frozen Section: A technique in which removed tissue is frozen, cut into thin slices, and stained for microscopic examination. A pathologist can rapidly complete a frozen section analysis, and for this reason, it is commonly used during surgery to quickly provide the surgeon with vital information.

Gland: An aggregation of cells (a structure or organ) that secretes a substance for use or discharge from the body.

Gland Volume: The size in cubic centimeters (cc) or grams of the prostate gland.

Gleason Score: A widely used method for classifying the cellular differentiation of cancerous tissue. The less the cancerous cells appear like normal cells, the more malignant the cancer. Two grades of 1-5, identifying the two most common degrees of differentiation present in the examined tissue sample, are added together to produce the Gleason score. High numbers indicate greater differentiation and more aggressive cancer. The grading system is named after its originator, Donald Gleason, M.D.

Globulin: Any of a number of simple proteins that occur widely in plant and animal tissues.

Gynecomastia: A side effect involving breast enlargement and tenderness, associated with various hormonal therapies that increase the level of estrogens in the body.

HDR brachytherapy: High Dose Rate brachytherapy involves the temporary insertion of radioactive iridium isotopes into the prostate gland using transrectal ultrasound guidance.

Hematuria: Blood in the urine.

Hereditary: Inherited genetically from parents and earlier generations.

Holistic Medicine: Medical care, which considers the patient as a whole, including his or her physical, mental, emotional, spiritual, social and economic needs.

Hormone: A substance produced by one tissue or gland and transported by the bloodstream to another to effect or regulate physiological activity such as metabolism and growth.

Hormonal therapy: Cancer treatment involving the blockage of hormone production by surgical or chemical means. Because prostate cancer is usually dependent on male hormones to grow, hormonal therapy can be an effective means of alleviating symptoms and retarding the development of the disease.

Hormone refractory prostate cancer: Prostate cancer that is androgen independent, and therefore, unresponsive to hormonal therapies.

Hot Flash: A side effect of some forms of hormonal therapy, experienced as a sudden rush of warmth to the face, neck, and upper body.

Imaging: Radiology techniques that are often computer-enhanced and allow the physician to visualize areas inside the body that would not normally be visible.

Impotence: See Erectile Dysfunction.

Incontinence: A loss of urinary control. There are various kinds and degrees of incontinence. Overflow incontinence is a condition in which the bladder retains urine after voiding. As a consequence, the bladder remains full most of the time, resulting in involuntary seepage of urine from the bladder. Stress incontinence is the involuntary discharge of urine when there is increased pressure upon the bladder, as in coughing or straining to lift heavy objects. Total incontinence is the failure of ability to voluntarily exercise control over the sphincters of the bladder neck and urethra, resulting in total loss of retentive ability.

Inflammation: Redness or swelling caused by injury or infection.

Informed Consent: Permission to proceed given by a patient after being fully informed of the purposes and potential consequences of a medical procedure.

Intensity Modulated Radiation Therapy (IMRT): The most recent state-of-the-art, computer-aided technique for delivering higher doses of radiation more accurately than either conventional External Beam Radiation or Conformal Radiation. The most advanced form of IMRT is Dynamic Adaptive Radiotherapy (DART).

Intermittent Androgen Deprivation (IAD): A temporary discontinuation of hormonal therapy that allows for a return to natural testosterone production in order to spare the patient from symptoms associated with androgen deprivation. Also referred to as Intermittent Hormonal Therapy (IHT).

Intravenous Pyelogram (IVP): A test that utilizes the injection of a special dye to check for injury or the spread of cancer to the kidneys and bladder.

Investigational: A drug or procedure allowed by the FDA for use in clinical trails, but not necessarily reimbursed.

Isodose Line: A line or two-dimensional shape that circumscribes an area receiving a radiation dose greater than or equal to a specified amount.

Laparoscopic Lymphadenectomy: The removal of pelvic lymph nodes with a laparoscope via four small incisions in the lower abdomen.

LH (Luteinizing Hormone): A chemical signal originating in the pituitary gland that causes the testes to make testosterone.

LHRH Analogs (or LHRH Agonists): Synthetic compounds that are chemically similar to Luteinizing Hormone Releasing Hormone (LHRH), used to suppress testicular production of testosterone. The most commonly prescribed LHRH analogs are Lupron® and Zoldex® Eligard® and Trelstar®. See also Luteinizing Hormone-Releasing Hormone (LHRH).

LHRH Antagonist: A chemical agent that blocks the LHRH receptor without the testosterone surge associated with

LHRH analogs. LHRH antagonists include Abarelix (Plenaxis®).

Linear Accelerator: A high energy x-ray machine generating radiation fields for external beam radiation therapy. These machines are typically mounted with a collimator (or multileaf collimator) in a gantry that rotates vertically around the patient being treated.

Localized Prostate Cancer: Cancer that is confined to the prostate gland, and therefore, considered curable.

Luteinizing Hormone-Releasing Hormone (LHRH): A chemical signal originating in the hypothalamus that causes the pituitary to make LH, which in turn stimulates the testicles to make testosterone.

Lymphadenectomy: The removal and examination of lymph nodes to precisely diagnose and stage cancer. See also Laparascopic Lymphadenectomy.

Lymph Node: A small, bean-shaped mass of tissue located throughout the body along the vessels of the lymphatic system. The lymph nodes filter out bacteria and other toxins, as well as cancer cells.

Magnetic Resonance Imaging (MRI): A painless, non-invasive technique using strong magnetic fields to produce detailed images of internal body structures. An MRI scan usually takes about 45 minutes per site.

Malignancy: A tumorous growth of cancer cells.

Malignant: Having the invasive and metastatic properties of cancer. Tending to become progressively worse and to result in death.

Margin: See Surgical Margin.

Metalloprotease Inhibitors: Drugs used to suppress the body's production of certain enzymes.

Metastasis: The spread of cancer, by way of the blood stream or lymphatic system, beyond the boundaries of the organ or structure where the cancer originated. Metastases is the plural. Metastatic refers to the characteristics associated with cancer that has spread or a secondary tumor.

Metastatic Work-Up: A group of tests, including bone scans, x-rays, and blood tests, to ascertain whether cancer has metastasized.

Monoclonal Antibody (mAb): An antibody that is directed against one specific protein (antigen).

Morbidity: Unhealthy consequences and complications resulting from treatment.

MRI: See Magnetic Resonance Imaging.

Nadir: The lowest point. Doctors sometimes use this as a verb to describe return of cancer or treatment failure. The PSA nadir refers to a minimum PSA value that should be maintained after treatment if the cancer has been successfully eradicated.

Necrosis: Death of cells or tissues caused by disease or injury.

Neoadjuvant: The use of a different type of therapy before primary, curative treatment. For example, neoadjuvant Androgen Deprivation Therapy is often used prior to radiation therapy or radical surgery, with the intent of improving the effectiveness of the primary treatment by reducing the size of the tumor and/or prostate gland.

Nerve-sparing: A procedure used during radical prostatectomy in which the surgeon attempts to save the nerves (neurovascular bundles) that allow for normal sexual functions.

Neurovascular Bundles: Strands of interwoven nerves and veins that run down the side of the prostate. The bundles contain microscopic nerves that are essential for erection; they also contain arteries and veins. Cutting the nerves in the bundles during surgery, or otherwise harming them in another procedure, usually renders the patient impotent.

Nocturia: Getting up at night to urinate.

Non-invasive: Not involving any incision in the body.

Oncogenes: Genes associated with tumor growth.

Oncology: The branch of medical science dealing with tumors. A medical oncologist is a specialist in the study of cancerous tumors.

Organ-confined Disease (OCD): Prostate cancer that is confined to the prostate capsule, as indicated clinically or pathologically.

Orchiectomy: A simple operation that involves surgical removal of the testicles, which produce most of the body's testosterone.

Osteoporosis: A decrease in bone mass and density causing fragility and porosity.

Overstaging: An assessment of an overly high clinical stage at initial diagnosis.

Palliative: Affording symptomatic pain relieve but not cure or remission.

Palpable: Capable of being felt when examined by touch or manipulation.

PAP: See Prostatic Acid Phosphatase.

Pathologist: A doctor who specializes in the examination of cells and tissues removed from the body.

PBRT: See Proton Beam Radiation Therapy.

Perineum: The area of the body between the anus and scrotum. A perineal procedure uses this area as the point of entry into the body.

Perineural Invasion: Describing cancer, which has spread from the prostate to the nerve bundles.

Periprostatic: Relating to the soft tissues immediately proximate to the prostate gland.

Photon: The quantum of electromagnetic energy, described as having zero mass and no electric charge. X-rays are high energy photons.

Placebo: A sugar pill often taken by participants in a medical study. Patients taking a placebo are compared to patients taking actual medications.

Ploidy Analysis: A pathological analysis to determine the number of sets of chromosomes in a cell.

Proctitis: Inflammation of the rectum.

Prognosis: A forecast of the course of a disease and future prospects of the patient.

Progression: A change in the status of the cancer indicating the condition has progressed and worsened.

Pro-oxidant: A term to describe substances that aid in oxidation.

ProstaScint® Scan: An imaging technique sometimes used determine whether or not cancer has spread to distant sites by using monoclonal antibodies.

Prostate Capsule: The outer membranous covering of the prostate gland.

Prostatectomy: The surgical removal of part or all of the prostate gland.

Prostate Specific Antigen (PSA): A blood test that measures a substance manufactured solely by prostate gland cells. An elevated reading indicates an abnormal condition of the prostate gland, either benign or malignant. It is presently the most sensitive tumor marker for the identification and monitoring of prostate cancer.

Prostatic Acid Phosphatase (PAP): An enzyme produced by the prostate that is elevated (3.0 or higher) in many patients when prostate cancer has spread beyond the prostate.

Prostatitis: An infection or inflammation of the prostate gland that is treatable with medications.

Proton Beam Radiation Therapy (PBRT): A form of radiation therapy that utilizes protons as the source of energy (as opposed to X-rays or neutrons).

PSA: See Prostate Specific Antigen.

PSA Bounce (or PSA Bump): A rise in PSA level after first having a reduction in PSA after radiation therapy.

PSA Nadir: The lowest PSA value after a particular treatment.

PSA Velocity (PSAV): The rate of increase of the PSA level, expressed as nanograms per milliliter per year.

Radiation Therapy (RT): The use of high energy rays to kill cancer cells and malignant tissue.

Radiation Urethritis: Inflammation of the urethra caused by radiation therapy.

Radical Prostatectomy: An operation to remove the entire prostate gland and seminal vesicles.

Radiosensitivity: The degree to which a type of cancer responds to radiation therapy.

RBA or Relative Biological Effectiveness: A scale used to compare the intensity of radiation associated with various atomic particles.

Receptor: A cellular docking site that interacts with a specific protein or enzyme (called a ligand). The interaction typically leads to the synthesis of other substances such as proteins, hormones or enzymes.

Recurrence: Return of the cancer following remission or treatment intended as curative. Local recurrence indicates a return of the cancer at the site of origin. Distant recurrence indicates the appearance of one or more metastases of the disease.

Refractory: A term indicating that the cancer no longer responds to the current therapy.

Remission: Complete or partial disappearance of the signs and symptoms of the disease. The period during which a disease remains under control, without progressing. Even complete remission does not necessarily indicate cure.

Resection: The surgical removal of a part of an organ or structure.

Risk: The probability that a particular event will or will not happen.

RP: See Radical Prostatectomy.

RT: See Radiation Therapy.

Rx: The standard abbreviation for prescription.

Salvage Treatment: A medical term for "Plan B." It means a patient must undergo another form of treatment because the first therapy was not successful. Salvage therapy may incur a higher rate of side effects.

Saw Palmetto: A nutrient extracted from the saw palmetto shrub, which is considered by some to aid the body's immune system.

Seed Implantation (SI): A minimally invasive procedure by which radioactive seeds are implanted into the prostate gland to destroy cancer. Also referred to as seeding and brachytherapy.

Selenium: A non-metallic element thought to be beneficial as a nutrient; it is often included in multivitamin supplements.

Seminal Vesicles: Glands that, like the prostate, support male reproduction. Fluid secreted by these glands regulates the consistency of semen.

Side Effect: A reaction to a treatment or medication, usually referring to an undesirable effect.

Sphincter: A circular muscle which contracts to close an orifice. The urethral sphincter squeezes the urethra shut, providing urinary control.

Staging: The testing process by which the extent and severity of a known cancer is evaluated according to an established system of classification. It is used to help determine appropriate therapy. See TNM Staging and Whitmore-Jewett Staging.

Surgical Margin: The outer edge of the tissue removed during a radical prostatectomy. The surgical margin may be "negative," indicating that no cancer is present and a better prognosis, or "positive," indicating that not all of the cancer has been removed.

Systemic: Throughout the body and affecting the entire body.

T-Cell: An immune system cell or lymphocyte that directs an immune response to malignant or infected cells.

Testes: Two male reproductive glands located inside the scrotum. The testes are the primary sources for testosterone. Also called testicles.

Testosterone: A male sex hormone chiefly produced by the testicles.

Thrombotic: Causing or relating to blood clotting.

TNM Staging: The most widely used classification system for evaluating the extent of prostate cancer. TNM refers to tumor, nodes and metastases. See Staging.

Transrectal: Through the rectum.

Transurethral: Through the urethra.

Transrectal Ultrasonography: See Ultrasound.

Transurethral Resection of the Prostate (TURP): A surgical procedure to remove tissue obstructing the urethra. The technique involves the insertion of an instrument called a resectoscope into the penile urethra, and is intended to relieve obstruction of urine flow due to enlargement of the prostate.

Tumor: An excessive growth of cells that is caused by uncontrolled and disorderly cell replacement. Abnormal tissue growth may be benign or malignant. See also Benign, Malignant.

TURP: See Transurethral Resection of the Prostate.

Ultrasound (Transrectal Ultrasonography): A painless, non-invasive diagnostic imaging technique using sound waves to create an echo pattern that reveals the structure of organs and tissues. It does not use x-rays.

Understaging: An overly low assessment of clinical stage at diagnosis.

Urethra: The tube that carries urine from the bladder and semen from the prostate out of the body through the penis.

Urologist: A physician who specializes in the diagnosis and the medical and surgical treatment of problems in the urinary and male reproductive systems.

USPIO: This technology uses ultrasmall superparamagnetic iron oxide (USPIO) as an MRI contrast agent for the identification of cancer metastasis in lymph nodes.

Vasectomy: A surgical procedure to render a man sterile by cutting the vas deferens, thus eliminating the passage of sperm from the testes to the prostate.

Vasoactive: Causing the dilation or constriction of blood vessels.

Vesicle: A small sac containing fluid, as in seminal vesicles.

Whitmore-Jewett Staging: A classification system for evaluating the extent of prostate cancer. This system is less widely used for the designation of stage than is TNM staging.

X-rays: High energy radiation that can be used at low levels of intensity to make images of the body's internal structures, or at high intensity for radiation therapy.

APPENDIX C

THE WARNING SIGNS OF PROSTATE CANCER

There are often no warning signs of prostate cancer. In some cases the following symptoms may indicate the presence of the disease. However, please be aware that these symptoms may also be due to benign conditions of the prostate, or other conditions entirely unrelated to prostate cancer:

- ✔ Elevated or rising PSA
- ✔ Abnormal Digital Rectal Exam
- ✔ Blood in urine
- ✔ Pain or difficulty urinating
- ✔ Increased urge to urinate, especially at night
- ✔ Hesitant or intermittent urinary flow
- ✔ Pain or discomfort in area of prostate
- ✔ Unusual and unexplained weight loss
- ✔ Continual pain in lower back, hips or pelvis
- ✔ Increased voiding urgency
- ✔ Inability to urinate
- ✔ Trouble having or keeping an erection (erectile dysfunction)
- ✔ Weakness or numbness in the legs or feet

ABOUT THE AUTHOR

Michael J. Dattoli, MD

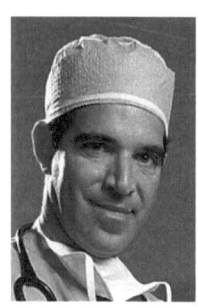

Michael J. Dattoli, MD, is a board-certified radiation oncologist with well over two decades of brachytherapy experience and has performed thousands of prostate implant procedures. He is considered the foremost pioneer in the field, optimizing brachytherapy designs to maximize tumor eradication and minimize symptoms. He has also been the leading trailblazer in the development of Dynamic Adaptive Radiotherapy (DART), utilizing all of the state-of-the-art modalities associated with 4-Dimensional Image-Guided Intensity Modulated Radiotherapy (3D-IMRT). Dr. Dattoli has successfully applied the same technologies to other forms of cancer, including breast, head and neck, GI, GYN, sarcomas and lung malignancies. He is a noted author and speaker in this complex field of medicine.

Dr. Dattoli attended the University of California at Berkeley and was the Valedictorian of his class at Vassar College; he earned his medical degree at Mount Sinai School of Medicine, Radiation Oncology at New York University Medical Center, then distinguished himself at Memorial Sloan-Kettering Cancer Center and New York Hospital-Cornell University Medical Center, as the Special Fellow in Brachytherapy. He was appointed Associate Professor in Brachytherapy and Radiation Oncology at Memorial Sloan- Kettering Cancer Center in New York and at New York Hospital-Cornell University Medical Center prior to relocating to Florida.

Dr. Dattoli also serves on multiple journal editorial review boards. Government appointments include "The Prostate Cancer Task Force" in Florida and consultant to the "Washington Oncology Roundtable Advisory Committee". He was selected by the International Association of Oncologists as a Leading Physician of the World and top Brachytherapist.

THE DATTOLI CANCER FOUNDATION MISSION

The Dattoli Cancer Foundation, sponsor of the Prostate Cancer Resource Network, is a 501(c)(3), tax-exempt charitable organization, whose mission is

◆ to raise awareness of the wide-spread incidence of Prostate Cancer and the need for early and annual screenings;

◆ to provide information and support to men newly diagnosed with Prostate Cancer as well as to those with recurrent Prostate Cancer, and

◆ to foster research into better diagnostic tools and treatment options for Prostate Cancer.

Gifts to the Dattoli Foundation make possible publications like this one, and are welcomed anytime. A copy of the official registration and financial information may be obtained from the Division of Consumer Services by calling toll-free (800-435-7352) within the state. Registration does not imply endorsement, approval or recommendations by the state.

Dattoli Cancer Foundation
2803 Fruitville Road
Sarasota, FL 34237
941/365-5599
800/915-1001
fax: 941/332-2317
www.dattolifoundation.org

ORDER MORE BOOKLETS IN THE SERIES

This *Prostate Cancer Essentials for Survival* booklet was prepared and distributed by the Dattoli Cancer Foundation, which is dedicated to providing information, hope and encouragement to prostate cancer patients and their loved ones. Additional booklets in this series are planned for publication in the near future. Previous titles include:

- ✔ *IMRT with DART and Brachytherapy*
- ✔ *Hormonal Therapy: Will It Benefit Me?*
- ✔ *The Dattoli Challenge: Evaluating Your Prostate Cancer Treatment Options*
- ✔ *Interpreting Your PSA: And Related Prostate Cancer Blood Tests*
- ✔ *Prostate Cancer Recurrence: Need You Be Concerned?*
- ✔ *Prostate Biopsy: When, Why And What To Expect*
- ✔ *Color-flow Doppler Ultrasound and Advanced Imaging for Prostate Cancer*

To find out when additional booklets will be released or to order copies of currently available booklets, please contact the Dattoli Cancer Foundation at (800) 915-1001.

www.ingramcontent.com/pod-product-compliance
Lightning Source LLC
Chambersburg PA
CBHW040247220526
45473CB00001B/400